YOUR KNOWLEDGE HAS VALUE

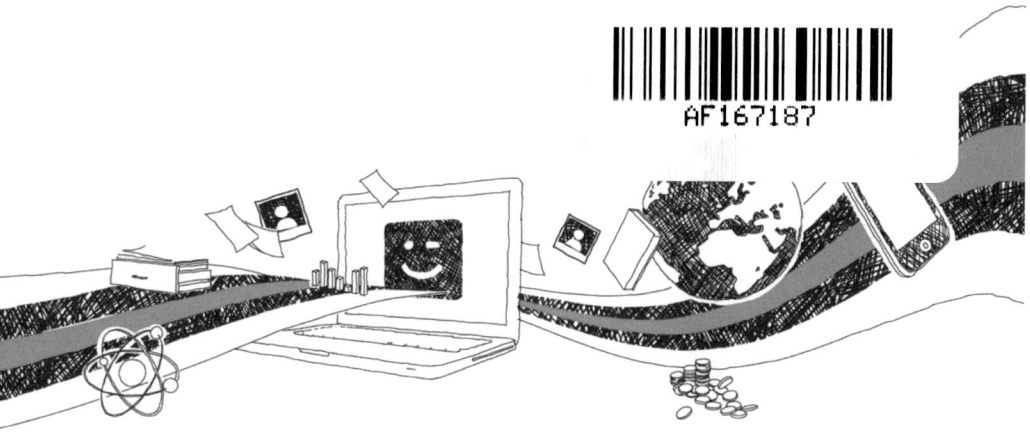
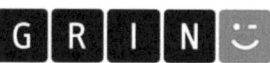

Chagas disease. Discovery of a TcGlcK inhibitor through lead optimisation of CBZ-GlcN

Maciej Nodzyński

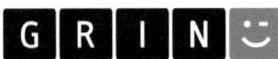

Bibliographic information published by the German National Library:

The German National Library lists this publication in the National Bibliography; detailed bibliographic data are available on the Internet at http://dnb.dnb.de.

ISBN: 9783346924865
This book is also available as an ebook.

© GRIN Publishing GmbH
Trappentreustraße 1
80339 München

Print and binding: Books on Demand GmbH, Norderstedt, Germany
Printed on acid-free paper from responsible sources.

The present work has been carefully prepared. Nevertheless, authors and publishers do not incur liability for the correctness of information, notes, links and advice as well as any printing errors.

GRIN web shop: https://www.grin.com/document/1381846

Discovery of a TcGlcK inhibitor through lead optimisation of CBZ-GlcN

Course: Medicinal Chemistry

Author: Maciej Nodzynski

Word count: 4129

Date: May 17, 2023

Abstract

Chagas disease, also known as American trypanosomiasis, is a neglected tropical disease that poses a serious threat to public health in South and Central America, but not only there. The disease affects large groups of people in underdeveloped areas, causing around 12,000 deaths every year. There is no effective treatment for the chronic phase of the disease, while the drug-resistant strains of the *Trypanosoma cruzi* parasite start challenging the usefulness of the acute phase treatment. Consequently, new drug candidates need to be developed. This paper proposes a novel drug candidate that was created by optimising the lead molecule called CBZ-GlcN. The affinity of the reported drug candidate is exceptional ($K_{diss} = 7.11$ nM), showing a 890-fold improvement over the affinity of CBZ-GlcN for TcGlcK. Furthermore, the new molecule exhibits advantageous pharmacokinetic properties. The paper also reports a suggested synthesis route for the drug candidate, which can be used to perform *in vivo* tests examining properties such as affinity, specificity, and toxicity of the drug candidate.

Introduction

Chagas disease, also known as American trypanosomiasis, is a parasitic disease that can be contracted mainly in South and Central America, which are the endemic regions. Although this disease was discovered over 100 years ago, only in 2005 did it get the attention of the public when WHO recognised Chagas disease as a neglected tropical disease (who.int, 2023). Since then, knowledge about Chagas disease has expanded and the treatment has improved, but still, it causes around 12 thousand deaths per year, with approximately 7 million individuals being infected at the moment (who.int, 2023). The disease concerns especially people in tropical and underdeveloped areas where access to medical care is limited, which makes the whole issue even more serious (who.int, 2023). Chagas disease is caused by a parasite called *Trypanosoma cruzi*, which uses triatomine bugs (also known as kissing bugs) as vectors (who.int, 2023). Triatomine bugs are nocturnal animals that feed on animals' blood, including humans, and that is how the disease can spread (who.int, 2023). It is enough if an insect bites the skin and leaves some feces (where the parasite is found) near the wound. Then, an individual may scratch their skin during sleep and transfer the feces with the parasite into the wound and bloodstream. Infected individuals can experience chronic health problems, such as heart disease and digestive tract problems, which can emerge even decades after the initial infection (paho.org, 2023). Chagas disease can result in death if left untreated (who.int, 2023).

Unfortunately, treatment options are limited. There is no vaccine for this disease, and the only antiparasitic drugs, benznidazole and nifurtimox, are most effective in treating acute cases when administered soon after the initial infection (who.int, 2023). They are less effective in treating chronic cases, whereas serious side effects often make patients quit the treatment before completion (Jackson, Y., Wyssa, B. and Chappuis, F., 2019). Additionally, Chagas disease is a silent condition, which means that the acute phase often goes without any symptoms or that the symptoms are present but are very general (who.int, 2023). Consequently, the disease can be easily mistaken for other conditions at an early stage, which may result in an individual not receiving appropriate treatment. As a result, it is beyond any doubt that Chagas disease is an unmet medical need. Especially the chronic phase needs to be addressed in order to tackle the disease in a more advanced and potentially life-threatening stage. New medications would also prevent the development of drug-resistant strains, which have already been observed and pose a serious threat to the effectiveness of the current treatment (Campos, M.C.O. et al., 2014). These issues have to be resolved as quickly as possible.

It is critical that the target protein is responsible for carrying out a process that is definitely essential for the parasite in order for a medication to be effective against most of *T. cruzi* strains. One of these processes is the catalysis of D-glucose to glucose 6-phosphate, which was recognised as necessary for the growth and differentiation of *T. cruzi* parasite cells (D'Antonio et al., 2015). As a result, *T. cruzi* glucokinase (TcGlcK) was identified as a target since the inhibition of this structure would significantly impair glucose synthesis and likely cause cell death. It should be mentioned that there is one more valuable target, which is T. cruzi hexokinase (TcHxK). It is present in higher amounts in the parasite and is also responsible for glucose synthesis; however, it cannot be taken into account since its crystal structure has not been determined yet (D'Antonio et al., 2015). Additionally, based on the comparison of secondary structures, the steric effects of TcHxK cause an unfavourable spatial arrangements of atoms when compared to TcGlcK, which would make it hard for the ligand to bind. Consequently, TcGlcK is a better target, and this will be shown even more when discussing receptor-ligand interactions (D'Antonio et al., 2015).

The complex of CBZ-GlcN and TcGlcK has been crystallized by Cordeiro, A.T. et al. in 2007 (PDB entry: 5BRE). D'Antonio et al. (2015) identified four potential inhibitors of TcGlcK, which can be seen in figure 1. These were Benzoyl Glucosamine (BENZ-GlcN), Carboxybenzyl Glucosamine (CBZ-GlcN), Hydroxyphenylopropyl Glucosamine (HPOP-GlcN), and Dioxobenzylthiophenyl Glucosamine (DBT-GlcN).

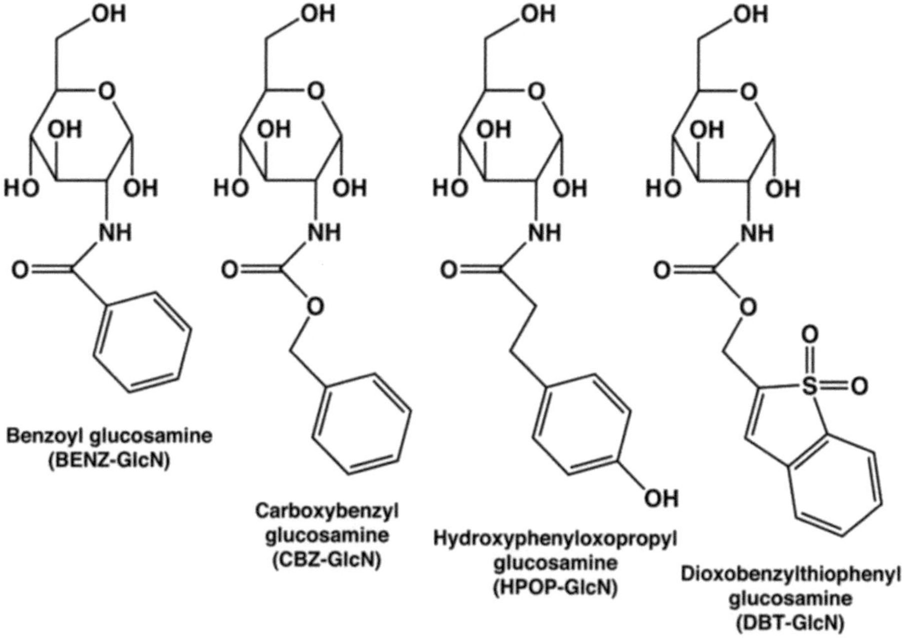

Figure 1: Names and chemical structures of four potential inhibitors for TcGlcK.

The finest inhibitor was determined to be CBZ-GlcN for a variety of reasons. Most importantly, it was crucial to make sure that CBZ-GlcN does not accidentally inhibit human hexokinase (HsHxKIV). HsHxKIV is also known as human glucokinase (HGlcK), and this term will be used from now on (Sternisha, S.M. and Miller, B.G., 2019). HGlcK is a human protein associated with absorbing and converting glucose (Sternisha, S.M. and Miller, B.G., 2019), whereas the ratio of dissociation constants between TcGlcK and HGlcK was equal to 246 (D'Antonio et al., 2015). Figure 1 shows that the phenyl group in the structure of CBZ-GlcN, while not the smallest, is definitely less bulky than the functional groups of other potential inhibitors, increasing the likelihood of effective binding. Additionally, it was discovered that CBZ-GlcN favours the beta anomer of the glucose moiety when binding to its active site (more precisely, affinity of CBZ-GlcN for the beta anomer is better), which is consistent with TcGlcK's preferred binding sites (D'Antonio et al., 2015). Binding is very likely to occur, and the active site of the hydrophobic pocket next to residue F337 is the optimal position for CBZ-GlcN (D'Antonio et al., 2015).

4

Methods

Affinity

All affinity-related computations were carried out using software called YASARA (Krieger and Vriend, 2014). Firstly, the crystal structure of TcGlcK in complex with the inhibitor CBZ-GlcN (PDB entry: 5BRE) was downloaded from the RSCB Protein Data Bank and imported to YASARA as a PDB file (Cordeiro et al., 2007) Afterwards, TcGlcK and CBZ-GlcN were separated and saved as two files titled 'receptor' and 'ligand', respectively (water was deleted). The ligand was subsequently docked locally to the receptor using Autodock Vina (Trott and Olson, 2009), which is a part of YASARA. A macro function called dock_runlocal.mcr was used to conduct local docking. The computed affinity of the lead compound was considerably higher than the value obtained by D'Antonio et al. (2015), (K_{diss} = 710nM). However, it must be taken into account that D'Antonio et al. (2015) determined the affinity under *in vitro* conditions, whereas YASARA gives only predictions based on elaborated algorithms. Consequently, neither the study nor YASARA can relate to measurements *in vivo*.

Many tries aiming to improve the affinity of CBZ-GlcN were carried out by removing and replacing groups that were shown by Poseview (Stierand and Rarey, 2007) to have no or little impact on the affinity. The replacement of groups was especially successful, and the best affinity was obtained through a sequence of single-point modifications. The affinity was computed by Autodock Vina after each change to track the influence of particular groups or atoms at particular locations on the affinity.

Selectivity

The binding affinity of the ligand to human glucokinase (HGlcK, PDB entry: 1V4S) was calculated in order to make sure that the optimised molecule (4UZO) is selective against T. Cruzi glucokinase and not human glucokinase (Kamata et al., 2004). The macro dock_run.mcr was used to dock the ligand (4UZO) globally to the receptor (HGlcK). As in the previous calculations, the affinity was determined using Autodock Vina. Additionally, global alignment of TcGlcK and HGlcK sequences was conducted to see the percentage similarity between these 2 proteins. A protein BLAST (blast.ncbi.nlm.nih.gov) was also carried out to see if there were any more off-targets the ligand might bind to.

The name '4UZO' was derived from the ligand residue name (4UZ) in the CBZ-GlcN-TcGlcK complex in the Protein Data Bank (PDB entry: 5BRE), while the remaining 'O' stands for 'Optimised'. This name will be used from now on.

Pharmacokinetics

Pharmacokinetic properties of the lead and optimised compound were computed mostly using SwissADME (swissadme.ch/index.php) and Marvin (chemaxon.com/calculators-and-predictors).

Moreover, when a particular intermediate showed a significant improvement in affinity, its pharmacokinetic properties were examined as well to see the direction in which they changed.

Synthesis

When the lead compound was successfully optimised, the retro-synthesis operation was carried out to establish the mechanism of the reaction that would lead to the formation of the optimised compound. The mechanism was determined using the program IBM RXN for Chemistry (rxn.res.ibm.com), whereas the program Chemdraw (chemdrawdirect.perkinelmer.cloud/js/sample/index.html) was used later to re-draw the mechanism and add annotations.

Results

Affinity

The affinity of the lead compound for the receptor was: $K_{diss} = 6331.33$ nM. Figure 2 presents the Poseview of interactions between the receptor (TcGlcK) and the lead molecule (CBZ-GlcN).The phenyl group of CBZ-GlcN interacts with the phenyl group of F337 through a π-stacking interaction in the active site of that pocket. It can also be seen that all OH and NH groups interact with the target molecule; however, there are also parts that seem to not contribute to the affinity. For example, the removal of a single-bonded oxygen and a carbon atom from the chain linking the two rings (-O-C-) might result in an increase in affinity. Additionally, the oxygen atom in the central ring also seems to be passive and could be replaced with a carbon atom to which other functional groups could be attached. Lastly, it can be examined what happens when OH groups from the central ring are replaced with more electron-donating NH_2 groups, since then it is expected that the hydrogen bonds will be stronger. With so many valuable interactions between the target and lead molecules, it is reasonable for the prospective medication made from CBZ-GlcN to also aim at the hydrophobic pocket close to residue F337 of the TcGlcK. There are several options for improvements that might be effective and result in a compound with better pharmacokinetic properties and greater affinity.

6

Figure 2: Poseview of interactions between CBZ-GlcN and TcGlcK. Dashed black lines show hydrogen bonds. Green lines show hydrophobic interactions, and green dashed lines show π-π interactions (Stierand and Rarey, 2007).

The whole optimisation process was done by applying the strategy of single-point modifications. Many intermediates have been obtained; however, only four were selected to be shown in the image below. All of the steps entailed a significant improvement in affinity (especially steps I, II, and IV), with some of them also having a positive impact on pharmacokinetic properties (especially steps III and V).

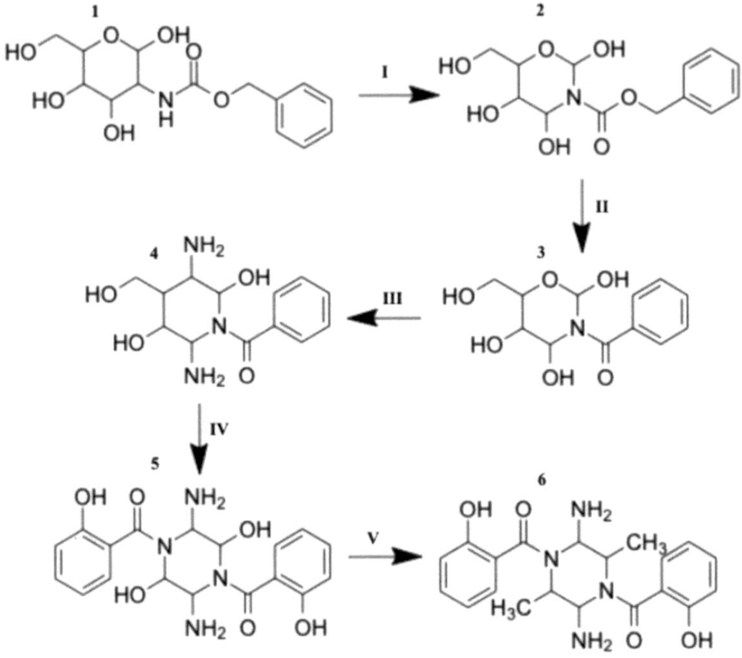

Figure 3: Overview of the optimisation process of the lead molecule CBZ-GlcN. In steps I, III, and IV, the major improvement was the affinity. Steps III and V involved also significant enhancements in the pharmacokinetic properties.

Figure 3 shows that in the first step, the N atom was shifted from the chain into the central ring, which improved affinity to 2200 nM. In step II, non-interacting C and O atoms were removed from the chain linking the two rings, which decreased the number of rotatable bonds from 5 to 3 and improved synthetic accessibility. Following that, step III involved the replacement of two OH groups with more electron-donating NH_2 groups and this action enhanced the affinity from 472 nM to 100 nM. Removing the oxygen atom from the central ring and adding one OH group also contributed to this effect. Step IV decreased the fraction of sp3 hybridised carbon atoms from 0.46 to 0.26, which was caused mainly by the addition of the second phenyl ring, which made the molecule more symmetric. Many significant improvements can be observed in the last step. The replacement of two hydrophilic OH groups with two hydrophobic CH_3 groups in the central ring decreased the polarity and increased LogP from 1.59 to 2.68. Additionally, all of the rules stated by Lipinski were respected since the mentioned replacement brought down the number of OH and NH_2

groups to acceptable limits (≤ 5). The last significant upgrade was that the gastrointestinal absorption (GI) changed from low to high.

Overall, the whole optimisation process was mainly about three sub-processes: 1). making the molecule symmetric, 2). replacing OH groups with either stronger (NH_2) or weaker (CH_3) electron-donating groups, and 3). shortening the chains linking the rings. When looking at figures 4 and 5, it can be easily seen that these were the main operations. The final product demonstrated excellent affinity with a K_{diss} of 7.11 nM, a 890-fold improvement compared with the lead molecule (K_{diss} = 6331.33 nM). The final molecule exceeded all of the previous intermediates, both in terms of affinity and pharmacokinetic properties.

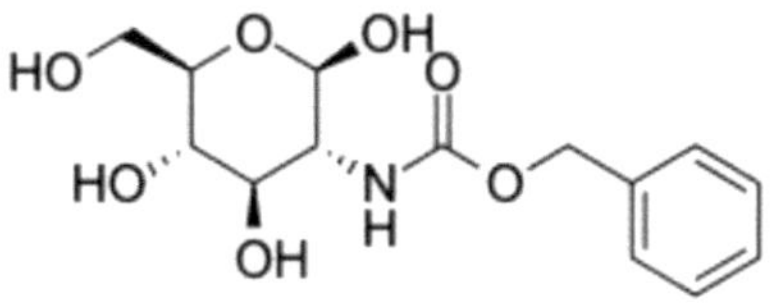

Figure 4: Two-dimensional structure of CBZ-GlcN, generated using ChemDraw.

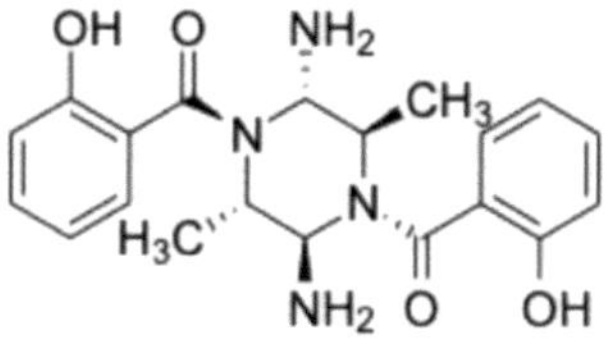

Figure 5: Two-dimensional structure of 4UZO, generated using ChemDraw.

The figures below present the Poseview of interactions between the receptor and the lead molecule (figure 6 - left), as well as between the receptor and the optimised molecule (figure 6 - right). Although the Poseviews look different at first sight, most of the original interactions stayed the same (e.g. Asp131A, Asn130A and Glu207A). The only valuable interaction that disappeared was the one between two phenyl rings, however, the other groups interact so nicely that this loss is not significant at all.

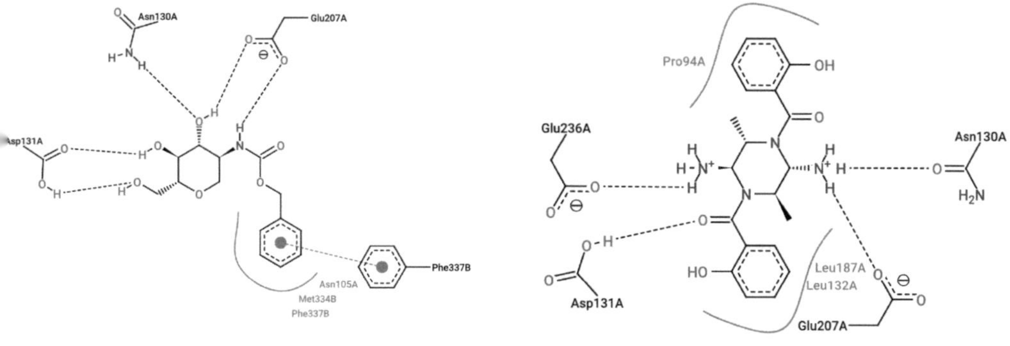

Figure 6: Right - Poseview of interactions between 4UZO and TcGlcK. Left - Poseview of interaction between CBZ-GlcN and TcGlcK. Dashed black lines display hydrogen bonds. Green lines show hydrophobic interactions, and green dashed lines show π-π interactions (Stierand and Rarey, 2007).

8

Selectivity

The BLAST analysis did not show any other significant off-targets, whereas the global alignment of TcGlcK (PDB entry: 5BRE, the ligand was deleted) and HGlcK (PDB entry: 1V4S) sequences showed 18% similarity. When 4UZO was docked to HGlcK, the following dissociation constant was obtained: K_{diss} = 3289.43 nM, which is far worse than the already mentioned affinity of 4UZO (K_{diss} = 7.11nM). As a result, 4UZO confirms the findings of D'Antonio et al. (2015), showing that it is species-selective.

Pharmacokinetics

The table below shows the pharmacokinetic properties of CBZ-GlcN (lead compound) and 4UZO (optimised compound).

Table 1: Pharmacokinetic properties of 4UZO compared with those of the original molecule, CBZ-GlcN. Most of the values were computed using SWISS ADME. *Values computed using Marvin Sketch, **The average from three docking operations.

Compound	CBZ-GlcN	4UZO
IUPAC name	2-benzoxyformamido-2-deoxy-hexopyranose	[2,5-diamino-4-(2-hydroxybenzoyl)-3,6-dimethylpiperazin-1-yl]-(2-hydroxyphenyl)methanone
Molecular weight	313.30 g/mol	384.43 g/mol
pKa*	11.68 (acid)	7.42 (base), 7.99 (acid)
LogP	1.41	2.68
LogD*	-0.88	2.20
GI Absorption	Low	High
Total Polar Surface Area	128.48Å²	133.12Å²
Num. rotatable bonds	6	4
P-glycoprotein substrate	No	Yes
Bioavailability	Yes, 0.55	Yes, 0.55
Lipinski's Rule of Five	Yes, no violations	Yes, no violations
Synthetic Accessibility	4.32	3.52
Affinity**	6331.33 nM	7.11 nM

The values of several parameters stayed the same even after the optimisation process. Firstly, and most importantly, good bioavailability was preserved while logP and logD values stayed within the acceptable range for the oral administration (Landry and Crawford, 2019). pKa values also remained within tolerable limits (Manallack, 2007). Other parameters, like total polar surface area and molecular weight, also remained similar, with 4UZO being slightly larger than the original compound. Moreover, both compounds comply with Lipinski's Rule of Five.

When it comes to differences, GI absorption has changed from low to high, which means that the optimised compound has a better permeability in the GI mucosa and, as a result, enters the bloodstream more easily. The optimised molecule has also become a P-glycoprotein substrate, which might be disadvantageous; however, the research on this topic did not state an explicit answer (Finch and Pillans, 2014). Additionally, the number of rotatable bonds decreased from 6 to 4, making the molecule more rigid. Synthetic accessibility has also changed from 4.32 to 3.52, which makes the molecule easier to synthesise. Lastly, an obvious improvement in the affinity was observed, which changed from 6331.33 nM to the excellent affinity of 7.11 nM. Overall, the pharmacokinetic properties of 4UZO are better than those of the lead molecule and, therefore, it is a promising candidate for becoming a drug for the chronic stage of Chagas disease.

Synthesis

The proposed synthesis route for 4UZO can be seen in Figure 7.

10

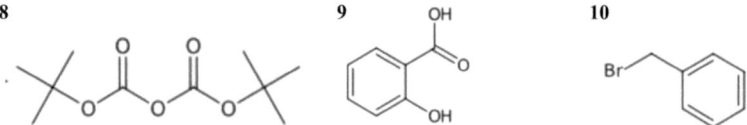

Figure 7: Proposed synthesis route for the synthesis of the optimised molecule, 4UZO. Compounds 8, 9, and 10 are commercially available additional reagents, which are di-tert-butyl dicarbonate ($C_{10}H_{18}O_5$), benzyl bromide (C_7H_7Br), and salicylic acid ($C_7H_6O_3$), respectively.

    The first step involved the reaction of compound 1 with compound 8, which resulted in protected NH groups which were previously exposed. It also created a part of the bridge between the central and future side rings. Afterwards, a substitution reaction took place, where the OH group was substituted with one phenyl group. It was done by carrying out the reaction of compound 2 with compound 9. The created compound resembled a mix of the lead compound and the final molecule. In step 3, substance 3 reacted with compound 9 to conduct N-acylation. Steps 4 and 5 involved the de-protonation of NH groups to become more electron-rich and therefore, more. nucleophilic. The last step involved the reaction with compound 9 to obtain a final product through the second N-acylation. It should be mentioned that compound 1 is not commercially available, and it may be a challenge to synthesise it. In the later stages of the mechanism, all compounds are either produced from the previous reaction or are commercially available.

Discussion

    A new drug candidate for the treatment of Chagas disease was introduced in this study. The emergence of drug-resistant *T. Cruzi* strains is calling for new medications against *T. Cruzi* parasites. T. Cruzi glocokinase (TcGlcK) was chosen as a drug target since its function is essential for the T. Cruzi parasite's survival. When calculated in YASARA, 4UZO exhibits extraordinary binding affinity ($K_{diss} = 7.11$ nM) to the TcGlcK enzyme. Compared to the binding affinity of the lead molecule (CBZ-GlcN), 4UZO shows an 890-fold improvement.

    SwissADME and Marvin were used to calculate the pharmacokinetic properties of both the lead chemical (CBZ-GlcN) and the medication candidate (4UZO). Both the lead compound and 4UZO have good pharmacokinetic properties and are anticipated to have sufficient bioavailability. Nevertheless, 4UZO is definitely a better molecule, both in terms of pharmacokinetic properties and binding affinity. While 4UZO appears to be a potential drug candidate, additional *in vivo* research is required to confirm its efficacy. Similar considerations apply to the lead molecule because the entire analysis conducted by D'Antonio et al. (2015) was performed *in vitro*.

    However, 4UZO needs to be synthesised first, and consequently, a synthesis route of TcGlcK was proposed. From there, it is possible to establish 4UZO's affinity for TcGlcK *in vivo*. The case of CBZ-GlcN has already shown that the values determined by YASARA can be very different from those obtained under *in vitro* or *in vivo* conditions; however, it is still anticipated that 4UZO will demonstrate improved affinity as compared to CBZ-GlcN *in vitro* and, most importantly, *in vivo*. Furthermore, *in vivo* research is necessary to show that 4UZO is not a toxic substance and that it penetrates the body sufficiently. Although pharmacokinetic properties indicate that 4UZO will not have any problems with bioavailability, more research *in vivo* is needed to confirm this.

It is also necessary to establish 4UZO's selectivity towards TcGlcK in comparison to other glucokinase enzymes. The drug candidate should not have significant binding affinity for the human glucokinase enzymes in order to avoid negative side effects. Docking of 4UZO to the human glucokinase enzyme revealed that the binding affinity was significantly worse (K_{diss} = 3289.43 nM) than that of 4UZO to the TcGlcK enzyme (K_{diss} = 7.11 nM). This means that 4UZO is very likely to have good species selectivity. However, this needs to be evaluated *in vivo*. Finally, it would be advantageous if 4UZO had an affinity for the TcGlcK enzyme found in other Trypanosoma species because this would suggest that 4UZO may potentially treat various types of trypanosomiasis. Then, 4UZO would be an even more promising drug candidate for the treatment of Chagas disease and other related conditions.

References

- Campos, M.C.O., Leon, L.L., Taylor, M.C. and Kelly, J.M. (2014). Benznidazole-resistance in Trypanosoma cruzi: Evidence that distinct mechanisms can act in concert. *Molecular and Biochemical Parasitology*, [online] 193(1), pp.17–19. doi:https://doi.org/10.1016/j.molbiopara.2014.01.002.

- Cordeiro, A.T., Cáceres, A.J., Vertommen, D., Concepción, J.L., Michels, P.A.M. and Versées, W. (2007). The Crystal Structure of Trypanosoma cruzi Glucokinase Reveals Features Determining Oligomerization and Anomer Specificity of Hexose-phosphorylating Enzymes. *Journal of Molecular Biology*, [online] 372(5), pp.1215–1226. doi:https://doi.org/10.1016/j.jmb.2007.07.021.

- D'Antonio, E. L., Deinema, M. S., Kearns, S. P., Frey, T. A., Tanghe, S., Perry, K., Roy, T. A., Gracz, H. S., Rodriguez, A., & D'Antonio, J. (2015). Structure-Based Approach to the Identification of a Novel Group of Selective Glucosamine Analogue Inhibitors of Trypanosoma cruzi Glucokinase. *Molecular and Biochemical Parasitology*, 204(2), 64–76. https://doi.org/10.1016/j.molbiopara.2015.12.004

- Finch, A. and Pillans, P. (2014). P-glycoprotein and its role in drug-drug interactions. *Australian Prescriber*, [online] 37(4), pp.137–139. doi:https://doi.org/10.18773/austprescr.2014.050.

- Jackson, Y., Wyssa, B. and Chappuis, F. (2019). Tolerance to nifurtimox and benznidazole in adult patients with chronic Chagas' disease. *Journal of Antimicrobial Chemotherapy*, 75(3), pp.690–696. doi:https://doi.org/10.1093/jac/dkz473.

- Kamata, K., Mitsuya, M., Nishimura, T., Eiki, J. and Nagata, Y. (2004). Structural Basis for Allosteric Regulation of the Monomeric Allosteric Enzyme Human Glucokinase. *Structure*, 12(3), pp.429–438. doi:https://doi.org/10.1016/j.str.2004.02.005.

- Krieger, E. and Vriend, G. (2014). YASARA View—molecular graphics for all devices—from smartphones to workstations. *Bioinformatics*, 30(20), pp.2981–2982. doi:https://doi.org/10.1093/bioinformatics/btu426.

- Landry, Matthew L. and Crawford, J.J. (2019). LogD Contributions of Substituents Commonly Used in Medicinal Chemistry. *ACS Medicinal Chemistry Letters*, [online] 11(1), pp.72–76. doi:https://doi.org/10.1021/acsmedchemlett.9b00489.

- Manallack, D.T. (2007). The pK(a) Distribution of Drugs: Application to Drug Discovery. *Perspectives in medicinal chemistry*, [online] 1, pp.25–38. Available at: https://www.ncbi.nlm.nih.gov/pmc/articles/PMC2754920/.

- Rcsb.org. (2010). *RCSB PDB: Homepage*. [online] Available at: https://www.rcsb.org/.

- Perkinelmer.cloud. (2019). *ChemDraw JS Sample Page*. [online] Available at: https://chemdrawdirect.perkinelmer.cloud/js/sample/index.html.

- Sternisha, S.M. and Miller, B.G. (2019). Molecular and cellular regulation of human glucokinase. *Archives of Biochemistry and Biophysics*, 663, pp.199–213. doi:https://doi.org/10.1016/j.abb.2019.01.011.

- Stierand, K. and Rarey, M. (2007). From Modeling to Medicinal Chemistry: Automatic Generation of Two-Dimensional Complex Diagrams. *ChemMedChem*, 2(6), pp.853–860. doi:https://doi.org/10.1002/cmdc.200700010.

- Swiss Institute of Bioinformatics (2022). *SwissADME*. [online] www.swissadme.ch. Available at: http://www.swissadme.ch/index.php.

- Trott, O. and Olson, A.J. (2009). AutoDock Vina: Improving the speed and accuracy of docking with a new scoring function, efficient optimization, and multithreading. *Journal of Computational Chemistry*, 31(2), p.NA-NA. doi:https://doi.org/10.1002/jcc.21334.

- www.chemaxon.com. (n.d.). *Marvin*. [online] Available at: https://chemaxon.com/marvin.

- www.rxn.res.ibm.com. (n.d.). *Homepage*. [online] Available at: https://rxn.res.ibm.com/.

- www.proteins.plus. (n.d.). *Zentrum für Bioinformatik: Universität Hamburg - Proteins Plus Server*. [online] Available at: https://proteins.plus/help/poseview [Accessed 10 May 2023].

- www.paho.org. (2023). *Chagas disease - PAHO/WHO | Pan American Health Organization*. [online] Available at: https://www.paho.org/en/topics/chagas-disease#:~:text=Chagas%20disease%20is%20considered%20a.

- www.who.int. (2023). *Chagas disease (American trypanosomiasis). [online] Available at: https://www.who.int/health-topics/chagas-disease#tab=tab_2.*

YOUR KNOWLEDGE HAS VALUE

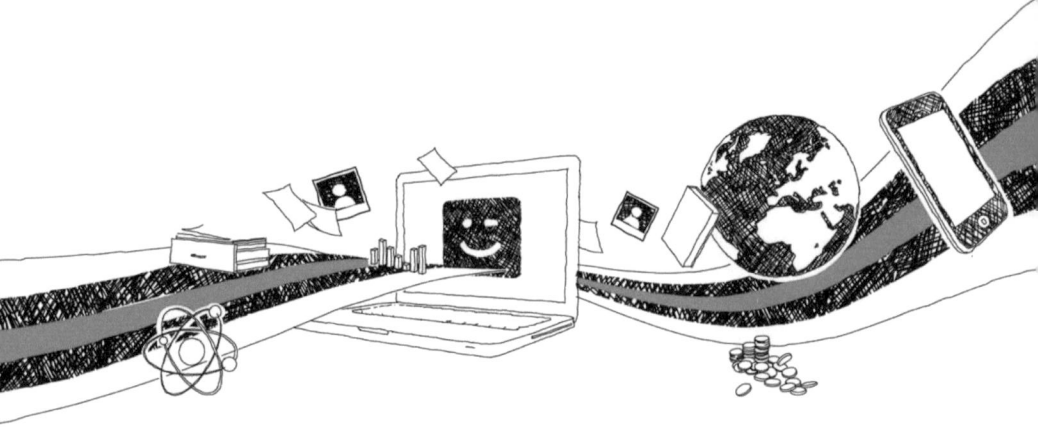

- We will publish your bachelor's and master's thesis, essays and papers

- Your own eBook and book - sold worldwide in all relevant shops

- Earn money with each sale

Upload your text at www.GRIN.com
and publish for free

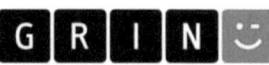